DIY REUSABLE FACE MASK PATTERN

Table of Contents
DIY REUSABLE FACE MASK PATTERN 1

INTRODUCTION 4
CHAPTER 1: BEST FACE MASK FOR VIRUS PROTECTION 5
1. Mask respirator 5
2. Face Masks disposable Co-power 6
3. Nuisance dust mask Honeywell, disposable 7
4. Medical Mask 3M N95 1860 8
5. Disposable mask 3layer breathable safety filter 10
6. Dynarex 2201 Medical-surgical face mask 11
7. Folding mask respirator SolidWorks 12
8. Kimberly-Clark mask Fluid Shield Procedure Face 13
9. 4530 universal heavy-duty non-toxic safety masks 15
10. Ellipse GVS SPR451 P100 Half respiratory mask 16
CHAPTER 2: EXAMPLE OF FACE MASK PATTERN 17
Material required for the first method 19
Disposables 21
CHAPTER 3: SOME ADVICE BEFORE YOU GET STARTED 23
I put in strong guard before spending time sewing masks: 26
CHAPTER 4: THE BEST MATERIALS TO MAKE A FACE MASK 27
For fabric loops, if you are not using elastic: 29
And if you cannot find elastic? 33
CHAPTER 5: HOW IS A CLOTH MASK USED? 37
Recommended products 39
Explanation 41
N95 masks must be appropriately fitted to work effectively 46
CHAPTER 6: PROBLEMS WITH A HOMEMADE MASK 50
Many risks associated with cloth masks 52

CHAPTER 7: WHY DO YOU NEED A FACE MASK FOR PROTECTION ANTIVIRUS? 58

CHAPTER 8: THERE IS ALSO THE N95 MASKS OR REUSABLE P100............. 60

CONCLUSION 64

INTRODUCTION

This project base on how to use and not to use a medical face mask. It we give more information base on the way to protect us from the virus and bridge the gap between human being and infection in the world.

The development of this face mask is to prevent or protect the human being from virus, and to overcome the challenges against this crisis, which have affected the standard of living and the world economy at large, and have impacted negatively.

CHAPTER 1: BEST FACE MASK FOR VIRUS PROTECTION

1. Mask respirator

First, this face mask 3M / N95 respirator certified by NIOSH (National Institute for Occupational Safety and Health). This means that it can effectively maintain particles larger than 0.3 microns. This is sufficient to block the water droplets carrying the virus.

I am pleased that this respirator/mask comes with a patented valve Cool Flow 3M. This helps to let out the heat and steam of my breath. He even helped keep the interior cool, dry mask. This infected mask also comes with a nose clip adjustable metal. This feature makes it easy to create a good seal around the face.

There are no loopholes that allow foreign particles to enter the inside of the nose and mouth. Braided elastic band provides sufficient rigidity to maintain the insured mask against my face. Fortunately, it's not so much that the cover will leave a mark on my skin when it comes out.

The problem I think most people, or at least most people have with this mask is that the elastic bands are tight. Fortunately, this is not so much that it becomes uncomfortable, but this oppression can sometimes be annoying.

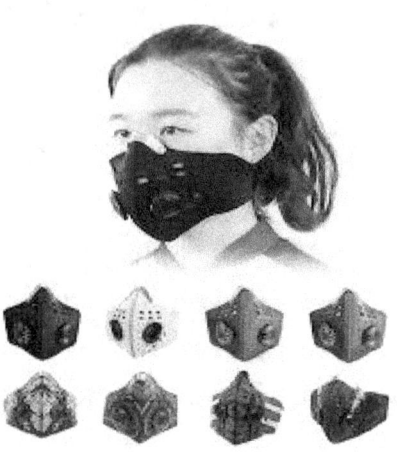

2. Face Masks disposable Co-power

Many people say that medical masks are not effective in protecting against viruses. However, putting two layers of tissue paper inside, this disposable mask may be helpful. One thing I liked about this the cover is that it is very cheap. For its reasonable price, you can get 100 pieces of throwaway masks.

Meanwhile, this mask can block particles that are greater than 2.5 microns wide. To give some perspective on how small it is, a human hair is 70 microns thick. Another thing to know about this mask is soft and comfortable it is to use. It is made of three layouts of non-woven material serving as the filter.

They are also soft to the touch. I can wear them without feeling any discomfort at all. I am also satisfied mainly because it comes with a metal clip on the soft nose. Simply clicking on the nose clip metal, you can create a good seal around the mouth and nose.

What little I have problems with is that this need not block the virus. If a person with the illness sneezes in the face, or at least, there is still a good chance of infection within three feet.

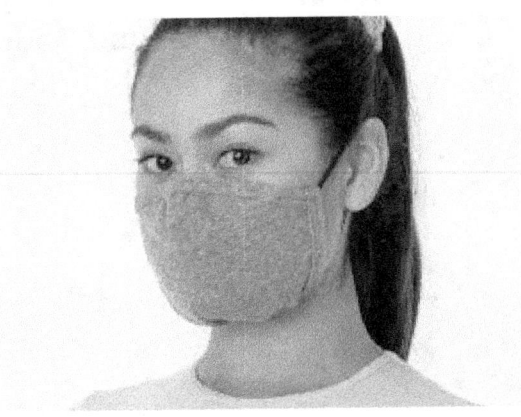

3. Nuisance dust mask Honeywell, disposable

NIOSH cannot approve this dust mask, so it has no rating, but they do an excellent job of filtering particles in the standard air. Although there is nothing that states if this is good to keep out illness, it is still managing than using nothing at all.

I like that the material is very soft. This allows it to fit comfortably against my face. They have no problem following the contours of the face. This mask also has a metal strip on the bridge of the nose.
You can tweak so you can clip onto your nose and create a good seal around the nose and mouth. fAt the beginning, I thought the single elastic band would not be enough to keep the cover in place, but when I tried it on, surprisingly clung quite well.

The biggest problem I have with this mask is that NIOSH does not approve cit, although it does a great job of blocking dust and odors certain chemicals, no way to know if it is effective against the virus.

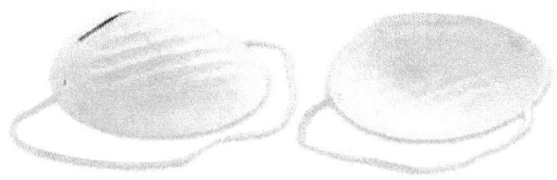

4. Medical Mask 3M N95 1860

Apart from being certified by NIOSH, this

surgical mask is also approved by the FDA as safe for medical use. These are classified as N95 to be filtered at the least 95% of all particles in the air, including most bacteria and viruses.

The little thing I like about this mask is that there is some foam padding on the metal nose clip. This provides some comfort and makes it bearable to wear the mask for hours.

The two elastic that goes over the head provide the right amount of elasticity to keep the mask firmly in place. Having two bands also helps distribute pressure evenly over the cover. This prevents twisting out of place after a while.

I am speaking of headbands, which are quite durable. I've been wearing these masks until the recommended time, and elastic bands do not loosen. What I do not like about this mask is that it has an exhalation valve. After a time, the heat that builds up inside the cover is placed a little too unbearable.

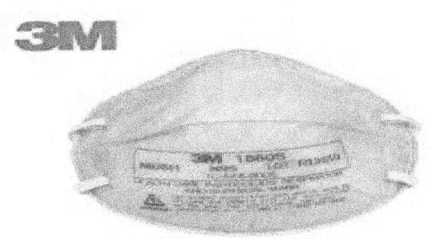

5. Disposable mask 3layer breathable safety filter

In the beginning, I was worried because these are simply generic surgical masks but perform very well. With some adjustment, these masks are capable of blocking foreign particles from reaching the nose and mouth.

The setting of this mask is also high. This is designed for an average adult face, and rubber bands are sufficiently flexible that they can even fit appropriately in young children. Moreover, if these are generic masks made in the US, He gave me some relief.

It pays to be selective with the spread of the virus as fast as it is right now. Moreover, even with all the panic going around, this mask is still being sold at a reasonable price while still having enough decent quality. The price is affordable and cheap for a day or two of breathing protection.

The only thing I do not like is that these are not branded. I have no qualms about using unbranded products, but they must have at least the name of the industrial on them to get attention to the customer later.

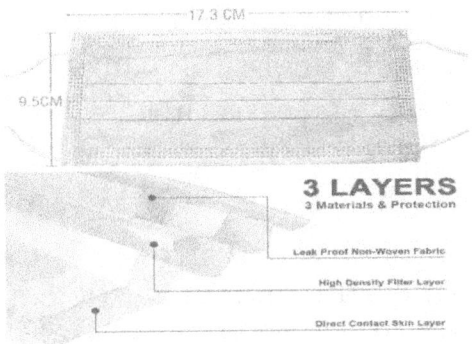

6. Dynarex 2201 Medical-surgical face mask

These masks are not classified N95, but they will do in a pinch. Many people say that these types of covers are ineffective, but in the absence of accurate particle filter masks, you can still be a great substitute.

Another reason I like this product is that it is very economical. You can get a modest amount of safeguards every day for just a low price, which is more practical than sick.
Although this product is affordable, note that this does not mean that loosens give adequate protection. This is made of medical-grade textile and can block more matter particles in the air.

The elastic bands also provide sufficient tension to hold the mask tightly pressed against the face without restricting breathing. The groups are also durable that could last a whole day.
I just have a problem with a face mask - and that's it's

a little too thin compared with similar products. Yes, it is quite possible that still can block particulate matter, but it is not so reassuring.

Although this is not an N95 respirator, if you are anxious about the virus, this will do fine in a pinch. You can do this merely sufficient by adding a couple of sheets of tissue paper. This will be infinitely better than not using any mask at all.

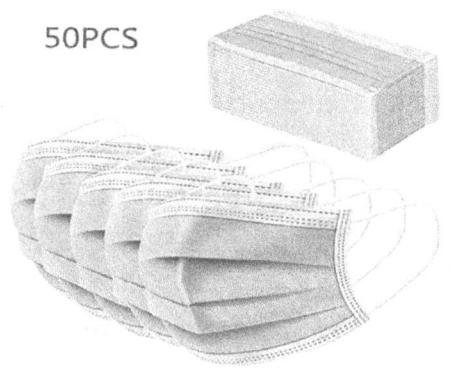

7. Folding mask respirator SolidWorks

I'm so impressed with this mask is having an exhalation valve. This helped keep the inside cool, dry cover, which is an issue that usually has simple surgical.

If you are doubtful, then I can assure you that this mask is NIOSH approved as an N95 respirator. This means that it can be locked at the least 95% of all particles, not based oil known suspension.

This also has a double layer of filter material

durable for optimum protection and durability. This product was initially destined as a dust mask used by craftsmen, so they need to be sustainable.

One thing about this mask is that it is very comfortable. Although it might seem rigid and hard, it adapts to the contours of the face and creates a seal around the nose and mouth.

The only problem I have with this product is that it is not on the list of approved N95 filtering masks CDC. This is not personally a big problem as many brands were not tested by the CDC but would have been better if this product was approved.

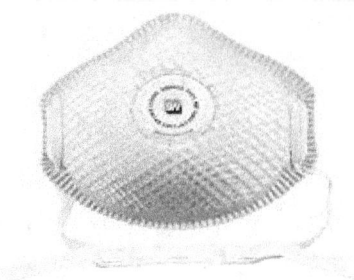

8. Kimberly-Clark mask Fluid Shield Procedure Face

The best of this medical mask is that it has the highest rating fluid resistance, which is level

3, as maintained by the American Society for Materials (ASTM).

I am delighted with this product because it came from one of the most reliable pharmaceutical companies worldwide, Kimberly-Clark. They will not risk putting their mark on any surgical mask.

A small detail that many might have overlooked is the small foam strip is placed in the metal nose clip. This small piece of foam provides a little padding that makes the mask a little more comfortable.

Another thing I liked is that this mask is soft and breathable. One would think that with the level of protection provided, the user would have to give up comfort, but it does at all.

The problem I have with these masks is not active. They work well. It's just that I realized they are so thin that it is difficult to convince myself of the product's efficacy.

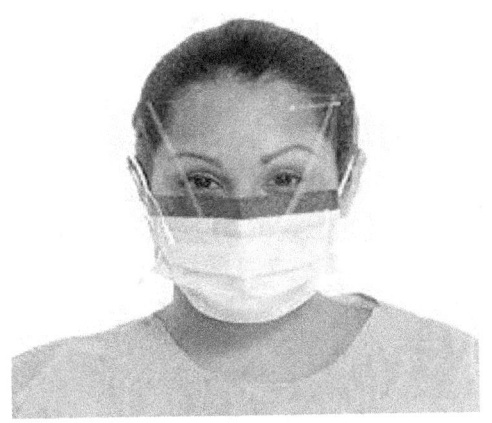

9. 4530 universal heavy-duty non-toxic safety masks

This mask is perfect for creating a good seal around the mouth and nose. In the beginning, I thought this is too hard, but when I gave one a try, I was surprised that it conformed to the shape of the face quite well.

I was also surprised at how light this mask is. After an hour or, I completely forgot that I was using it. The cover has a metal band placed around the nose. When pressed against the nose, the group will bend and form around the bridge of the nose, creating a good seal around them at all.

The issue I have with these masks is not valid. They band, but strong and elastic. The group has sufficient elasticity to keep the flat mask against his face securely, but not so tight that it is uncomfortable. There is a problem with these masks. N95 masks are not NIOSH approved. This could discourage some of these respirators, even giving it a chance.

Although this mask is NIOSH approved, if you are in a bind, it will work better than just using a tissue to cover your mouth. Also, these masks N95 could be equivalent (at the least in my experience, they seem to be).

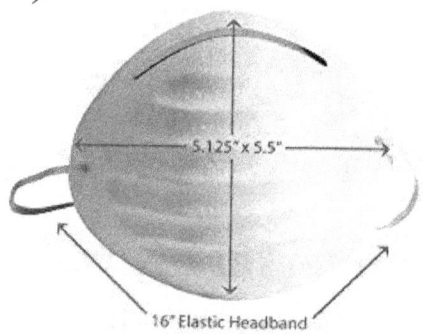

10. Ellipse GVS SPR451 P100 Half respiratory mask

The best feature is that this respirator is NIOSH approved and classification of P100. This means that it can filter nearly 100% of all particles suspended in air, including chemicals-based oil.
The N95 respirator is 100% silicone, which means it is completely hypoallergenic and adorable. You can make a complete seal around the nose and mouth. Nothing can get inside the mask.

They were speaking of the filters if it is not used for construction purposes, which It can be used for a week to a month. Simply replace the cleaners when they get too clogged with dust.
The mask also has an exhalation valve pointing downwards. What those means is that you are

wearing glasses that do not fog whenever you breathe out. This also keeps the interior dry and cool mask.

Protective masks are essential when it is likely that work carried out to discard the dust, vapors, gases, and other toxic products ... To protect adequately, models can use a single-use disposable or reusable models adapted to each situation. You still have to know how to recognize them, choose them, and use them!

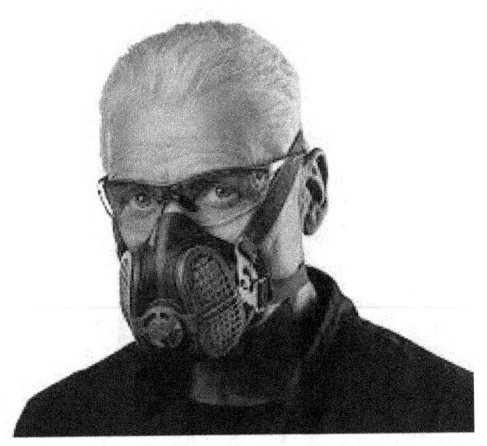

CHAPTER 2: EXAMPLE OF FACE MASK PATTERN

Several easy-to-make options exist to cover your face with your creation. These alternatives will allow the masks of procedures and the famous N95 to be left to health professionals who are at higher risk.

Seamless

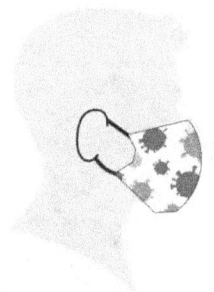

Even if you don't know how to sew, you can still make masks at home. They may be less comfortable and aesthetic than those with seams, but they are always convenient.

The easiest way is to fold a square piece of fabric and slip rubber bands at the ends of the rectangle you will get, If you have a t-shirt that you no longer wear, you can cut out a mask that you will attach behind your head.

Material required for the first method

- Fabric square
- Hair elastic, elastic cords or rubber elastic

Material required for the second method

- An old t-shirt
- A good pair of scissors

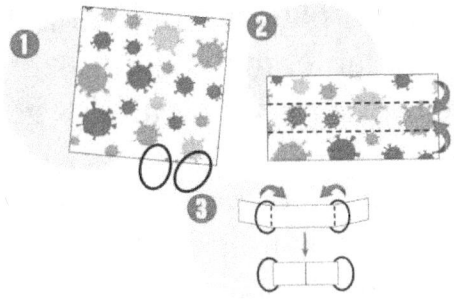

Steps

1. Start with a piece of fabric and two hair ties.
2. Place a paper towel in the center of the material then fold the top and bottom of the fabric over the paper towel.
3. After sliding the elastic bands, wrap the sides of the fabric towards the center by inserting one hand into the other before placing it on your face.

Sewn masks

Do you own a sewing machine, or do you know how to use a needle? You can start designing a sewn mask. Several patterns and tutorials that vary in difficulty are available, including this one. Besides, it is not forbidden to let your creativity go by changing the fabrics.

The simplest and most effective option is a rectangular mask with folds to better cover the nose and chin. If you do not want to sew, it is still possible to use fabric glue or diaper pins to hold everything in place; however, this could affect comfort.

Material required:

- Fabric, preferably cotton
- A sewing machine or needle and thread
- Scissors
- Elastic cords or fabric straps
- It is also possible to obtain kits, including all the necessary material on the web. The company Club Tissus sells sets allowing the production of five masks. For each sale, $ 3 will be donated to the Chaînon, an

accommodation resource for women in difficulty in Quebec.

Disposables

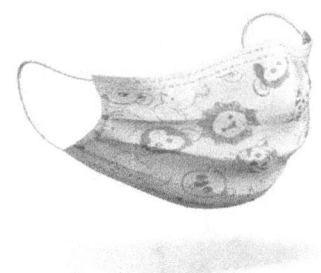

Disposable masks, although less ecological, do not need to be maintained, unlike those made of fabric. Note, however, that health authorities do not recommend them. Researcher Geneviève Marchand of the Robert-Sauvé Institute also raises a caveat about very absorbent materials that can release the liquid after a certain period.

The method for making them resemble those of fabric. First, superimpose two sheets of absorbent paper which you will fold into an accordion.

Place rubber bands at the ends and fold them back on themselves. Hold everything with staples or sticky paper.

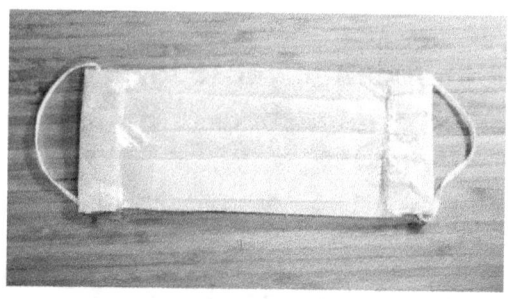

You can add a coffee filter to the side that will touch your face by holding it in place with staples.

Material required

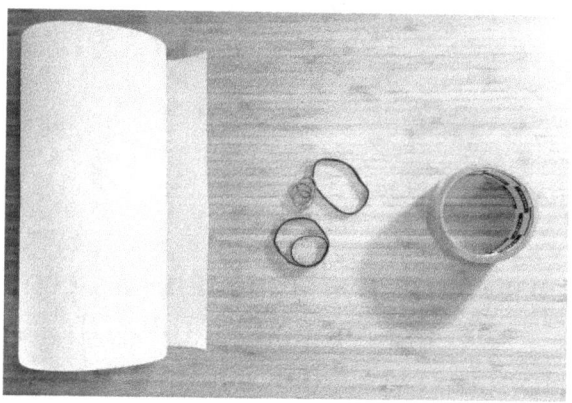

- Absorbent paper
- Coffee filter
- Stapler
- Rubber elastic

Fabrics to cover the face

If you do not want to tinker, it is possible to wear a scarf, a neck warmer, or a bandana to cover the face. However, these accessories are more likely to slip and may need to be replaced, which will result in hand-to-face contact.

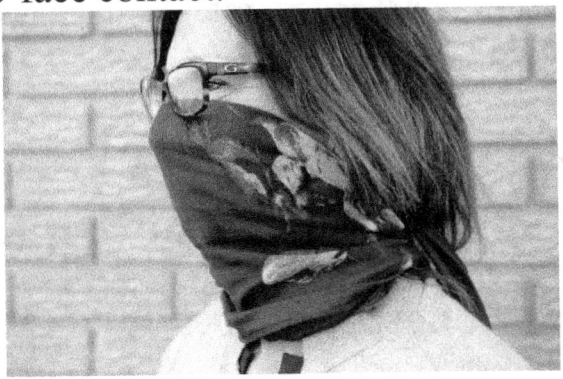

CHAPTER 3: SOME ADVICE BEFORE YOU GET STARTED

The public health maintenance of Canada has some recommendations for the design of non-medical masks. They must:
- ➤ Be made up of at least two layers of fabric (such as cotton or linen)
- ➤ Cover mouth and nose entirely without leaving holes
- ➤ Be securely attached to the head by ties or cords forming loops that go behind the ears.
- ➤ Allow easy breathing
- ➤ Be comfortable and wear without requiring frequent adjustments.

- Be changed as soon as possible if they become wet or dirty.
- Keep their shape after being washed and dried.

DIY facial masks are not as effective as surgical masks authentic.

Is there a need for cloth face masks?

Currently, the supply of surgical masks is the lowest of all critical times nationwide. Orders for standard disposable masks used in hospitals are ordered around, and there is a great demand for protective equipment for health workers. According to the CDC, cloth masks are an option for responding to crises when they have exhausted other supplies.
Because of these concerns, many hospitals across the country have requested surgical masks made at home as a temporary emergency measure.

The CDC now recommends using face cloth coatings.
Also, federal health officials now recommend that people's mouth and nose with cloth masks are covered in public.
This is a voluntary public health measure to curb the spread of help when people need to visit public places such as grocery stores and public transport

stations.

CDC also advises using pure fabric coatings to reduce the spread of the virus and help people who may have the illness and do not know to transmit it to others.
Sewing a fabric mask to be allowed medical surgical masks and N95 masks degree are professionals and patients' health care reserved.

An important distinction

homemade masks are not as effective as an N95 filter mask
Instead, they are intended:
To meet the demands of covers in emergency hospitals.
Community members help "curb the spread" in public places where other social distancing measures are challenging to maintain.
Sources Readings: Cambridge study, Nature, occ. Approx. Med, Annals Occ Health)

Face masks are home the Last haunt

The Centers for Virus Control and Prevention (CDC) said that in times of crisis, homemade masks are acceptable as a last resort. On the CDC website, strategies to optimize the supply of face masks explain that if homemade face masks are not a substitute for the PPE, it can be used in situations where facemasks are unavailable.

HCP use homemade masks:

In places where facemasks are unavailable, HCP can use homemade masks (e.g., bandana scarf) to treat patients with Covid-19 as a last resort. However, homemade masks are not considered PPE. For their protection capacity, HCP is unknown. One must be careful to find this option. Homemade masks should ideally fabric be used in combination with a mask that covers the entire front (which extends to the chin or below) and the side of the face.

I put in strong guard before spending time sewing masks:

Follow CDC guidelines as the situation evolves.
Contact your local clinic and hospital to ensure they accept masks, masks, and all that you will meet their guidelines.

Some hospitals require surgical masks homemade.

Some hospitals and clinics that accept donations of homemade masks. Organizations such as masks for Heroes now have a facility database in search of gifts. If you are wondering where you can mask help, a hospital or clinic needs to donate found, to make a big batch of masks sewing donations before spending time, please ask first if they accept.

You should ask if this model (2 layers of fabric with a pocket for additional disposable inserts) will meet their needs. You should also ask about the procedures of landing/pickup.

CHAPTER 4: THE BEST MATERIALS TO MAKE A FACE MASK

scientist at Cambridge University has tested the usefulness of a wide range of household materials in homemade costumes. They measured how domestic materials could capture and filter small particles.

The test data shows that the best choice for DIY fabric masks is cotton T-shirts, pillowcases, cotton, or other materials. Using a double layer of content for your DIY mask adds a small increase in filtration efficiency.

Other research has found that the most effective two layers masks heavyweight "quilters cotton" thread density at least 180 were constructed, and it was one more tight thicker tissue.
This pattern has two layers of fabric and an inner bag

in which one can add layers of disposable filter material if desired.

materials for a fabric hospital mask
The DIY surgic

pins or clips al mask pattern

- ➤ The finished mask adult is 7.75 "wide and 3.75" tall.
- ➤ materials
- ➤ 100% cotton fabric (with a tight weave)
- ➤ 1/8 "flat elastic loops for ear loops, or four fabric (can use the same woven fabric to strips, using pre-made bias or strips cotton knit)
- ➤ fabric scissors

sewing machine and thread

Cut List

- For a mask adult size:
- Cut one material rectangle 16 "long and 8.5" wide
- Cut two pieces of elastic, each 7 "long (or even 8" for adult size)
- For a small child-sized mask:
- Cut one fabric rectangle 14 "long and 6.5" wide
- Cut two pieces of elastic, each 6 "long

For a large infant size mask:

- Cut one rectangle fabric 15 "long and 7.5" wide
- Cut two pieces of elastic each 6/5 "long

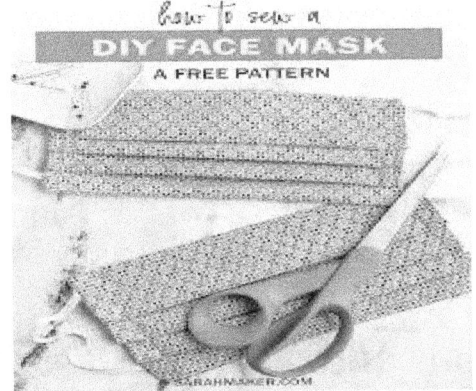

For fabric loops, if you are not using elastic:

Cut four rectangles 18 "long by 1.75" wide. Fold long sides to meet in the middle and fold in half again to enclose the raw edges cosa down the length of the rectangles along the edge to create the loops.
18 "for some people may be too long, especially children.
diagram showing how to sew cloth masks for hospitals

Step 1: Sew on the upper side, with pocket.

Fold the cloth rectangle in half, with the right side against the other.

Sew along the top 8.5 "wide edge, using a large 5/8" seam allowance. Leave a hole 3 "-4" in the center of this seam to create an opening for the pocket filter, and to allow the mask is right side out after sewing. In the image above, I have marked this opening pins.

Update: Some people find it easier to insert/remove the additional filter if they make a larger opening. Instead of a 3-inch opening left "opening, you could make a 4".

materials and supplies to sew a surgical mask

I do not want a pocket filter? If you do not want or need a pocket, that's fine. Anyway, you will have to leave an opening so you can rotate the mask right out. After connecting the elastic or ties (in the next step) and the right cover turned out, you can see the closed opening. Then you can continue with the rest of the directions, sewing seam meter fabric filter surgical mask then turn the fabric so that the seam of the opening of the pocket is centered in the middle of one side. Using an iron, press the seam open.

Fold the excess margin seam under which encloses the edge of the fabric weave. Topstitch or zigzag along each side of the seam to finish the edge. This will help keep the fabric fraying to the insert and remove any filter.

Step 2: Elastic Pin or gender Ties If used elastic:

Pin a piece of elastic to each side of the mask, one end to the top corner and one end to the bottom edge of the rectangle of the fabric. This will create the ear hook once the cover is on the right side out and pleating. Placing the ends of the elastic about 1/4 "to 1/2" from the top and bottom corners of the fabric.

The elastic piece itself is sandwiched between two layers of fabric. Once you turn on the right side of the mask, the elastic is abroad.

Repeat to make this process on each side two loops ear.

Using tissue fasteners - Alternative:

If you cannot find elastic or prefer using fabric links, you can use four fasteners fabric, one in each corner. Each tie is 18 "long. Sew one lace in each turn, being careful not to catch the links in the side seams.

You can also use the twill tape, bias tape, or strips of cotton jersey (shirt fabric).

The finished mask will then be carried by attaching the fabric that remains behind the head. See notes at the end of the post.

Step 3: sewing the sides, fixing links with a

seam allowance 3/8 ", sew each side of the face mask. Backstitch on the elastic ties or fabric to secure them. Cut corners with scissors so that it will be easier to turn the cover on the right side Be care not to clip the stitches coincidentally.

Turn the mask right side out and press with an iron. You can use a pencil to push the corners using a wire to create a flexible nosepiece to a fabric mask

Optional: Insert an adjustable nose piece Cut a 6-inch piece of pipe cleaner, floral wire, or other flexible wire to create a nose piece. I folded the rear ends of the son in to prevent them from poking through the fabric. Place the wire through the hole pocket and slide it to the top of the mask. Assembly around on three sides to hold it in place.

Step 4: Folds Make the mask with three evenly spaced lines. To do this, you can measure and mark with a fabric pen water-soluble. Or, you can do what I did, and bend the mask quarters - fold the sides to meet in the middle and again fold in half. Use an iron to make a crease, use pins to secure three plies on a surgical mask fabric.

Use your brand to create three evenly spaced 1/2 "folds. Pin the folds down, make sure that all folds are in the same direction. Sew along the sides to fix the creases. I love to sew the sides twice, just to be sure.

When the mask is worn, pleats are open downwardly

to prevent the collection of particles in the folding pockets sewing folds down onto the side of a surgical tissue mask for hospitals Troubleshooting pattern

And if you cannot find elastic?

I heard many people who are struggling to find elastic. If you cannot find flexible to earrings, you can make a mask with fabric fasteners instead. You can use ready-made 1/4 "twill tape, double-fold bias tape, or cut long strips of fabric of cotton tightly woven that you use for the rest of the mask.

For links through fabric: Cut 18 "long strips of cloth, 1.75" wide. Fold long sides together (the length of the hot dog style), so they meet in the middle. They were then folding the strips to one and one-half (range) to wrap the raw edges. Point down the pieces along the side to create links.

how to make strips of bias binding tissue

If you want these straps for a bit of stretch, you can cut long pieces of cotton jersey or knitted material t-shirt. The great thing about using jersey fabric is that it forms a tube when you stretch. And, it is comfortable to wear, as it keeps a little stretch.

Whichever option you choose, you'll want to cut four pieces approximately 18 "long and tie a band at each corner. The mask secures by attaching the straps behind the head.

What metal to help the adjustment to better mask?

To help the mask fit better around your nose, you can insert a length of flexible metal inside the top of the cover, through the insert pocket opening before forming the folds. Then you can topstitch down around the surgical metal insert to keep it in place. I have seen people use pipe cleaners, floral wire, or fasteners.

What can be used as a filter?

It is so important that everyone understands that while using a cloth mask can provide some level of protection, cannot protect against viruses in the same way an N95 mask can.

Many different types of filters have been suggested, such as coffee filters, felt, and vacuum filter bags. Not all of these filters are effective, and not all of them are safe.

Without further research on the safety and effectiveness of materials filter face mask, we will not know what

It is the best filter.

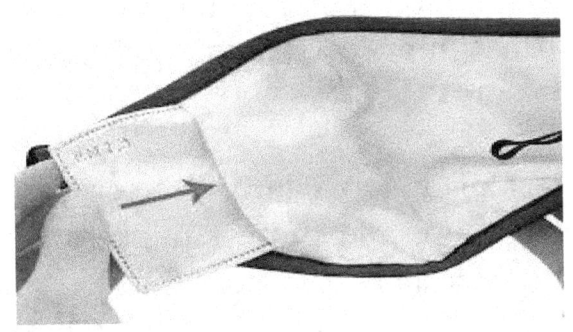

Facial mask filter materials: pros and cons

HEPA filters. In tests, a layer of HEPA vacuum cleaner bag seemed to perform the best. However, it is difficult to breathe. Many people have expressed concern about the safety of materials (such as fiberglass) used to produce these filters. Right now, I cannot recommend it.

Coffee filters. One of the designs masks the CDC has published a layer of a coffee filter. They are readily available and disposable.

Blue shop towels. Others have tested the effectiveness of blue sheets workshops like this. They are promising, but the data have not been released publicly or verified.

Dryer sheet or baby wipes. Because these elements are covered with fragrances and other chemicals not recommend the use of these as a filter.

Non-woven interface.

Flannel or felt. These materials are not as tightly woven cotton fabric as outside the mask, so it is doubtful that improve efficiency filtration. Also, it can trap moisture.

A layer of cotton fabric. We research suggests that a more secure and more straightforward option for a filter material is a cotton shirt or cotton cloth tightly woven, If you are sewing for hospitals that may have their medical-grade filters, always call before sewing to check your requirements.
Disclaimer: This pattern has not been tested in the industry and is intended for educational purposes only. The decision to use this device is the only of its own.

Where can you donate masks?

Not all hospitals are requesting masks, but many are. Find your local hospital to see if they have asked for donations.
Many groups, such as sewing and craft Alliance, are working to connect volunteer sawists health organizations and registering.

Also, an organization called Masks for Heroes has a website with a database of facilities currently looking for donations. If you are wondering where you can donate masks, which can help find a hospital or clinic that needs them.

CHAPTER 5: HOW IS A CLOTH MASK USED?

It is essential to use the proper procedures for donning and doffing his mask. Be careful not to touch your eyes, nose, and mouth when the cover is removed and wash your hands immediately afterward.

Here is a clear step by step guide to the best way to properly wear a face mask.

Important note: the CDC, masks "should not be placed in young children under two years old who has trouble breathing or is unconscious, incapacitated, or unable to remove the cover without help."

How to clean and disinfect cloth mask?

Only use dry masks when they get wet covers, even if only from breathing, which needs to be cleaned.

Masks regularly wash with detergent and regulate the machine cycles hot wash. Dry completely.

DIY fabric Surgical mask

Homemade cloth surgical mask to be

worn as a last resort in a crisis.

Materials

- cotton fabric, tightly woven
- 1/8 "elastic cords, or fabric
- Tools
- sewing machine and thread
- the scissors

rule

pins or sewing clips

Instructions

Cut the fabric. For an adult-sized mask, cut one rectangle of fabric 16 "long and 8.5" wide. Cut two elastics, each 7 "long. Or, cut four fasteners fabric 18" long.

For a mask size child, cut one rectangle of fabric 14 "long and 6.5" wide. Next, cut two pieces of elastic, each 6 "long. I am sewing the upper side with a pocket opening. Fold the fabric in two, with the right-side face.

Sew along the 8.5 "wide edge using an 8/5" seam allowance. Leave a 3 "opening at the center of the seam to create an opportunity for the filter sock, and to enable the mask to be rotated to the right after sewing.

Sewing along both sides of the seam of a sharper

edge.

Pin elastic fabric or tie. Pina flexible member on each side of the mask, from one end to the apex angle and one end to the corner of the bottom. If you use cloth ties, pin a knot at each corner, with the rest of the knot sandwiched inside two layers of fabric.

Sew side. Sew the hands of the face mask backstitch on the elastic ties or fabric for secure.

Cut corners, turn right on the mask, and press with an iron.

Sew Pleated

Create three evenly spaced 1/2 "folds. Pin the folds in place, making sure all the creases are in the same direction. Sew each side to secure the folds.

Note: when the mask is worn, pleats are open downwardly to prevent the collection of particles in the folding pockets.

Some hospitals are applying for an opening of the large pocket for filter changes faster - 4 "deal.

For a small size child, start with a square that is 6.5 "by 14".

For a big kid size, start with a square that is 7.5 "by 15."

Recommended products

Colour scissors sewing pins 250 pieces of glass ball quilting pins Headpins jewelry decoration dressmaker

Brother Quilting Machine, CS7000i, 70 stitches built

2.0 "LCD screen, table width, including ten sewing feet.

Brother Quilting Machine, CS7000i, 70 stitches built 2.0 "LCD screen, table width, including ten sewing feet.

Dritz 9330W braided elastic, White, 1/4 inch by 3-Yard

He did this project?

A free pattern for sewing surgical masks home for hospitals. Make a pleated mask series with a filter pocket and elastic ear loops or loops woven fabric or cotton T-shirt material.

Remember, before you start sewing a massive lot of masks, please call the hospital or clinic and make sure you both want and can accept homemade masks.

This week, give it to Dr. Hoda Kardooni again, which investigated the science behind medical masks, respiratory masks, N95 masks, and fabric. As highlighted in this article, you will discover strict protocols to follow if you want a cover to work effectively.

There is much debate in progress on a face mask for public use. At this challenging time, it is understandable that people are desperately looking for anything that can help protect against the pandemic however vaguely either using the mask or believe the assertion of any news agency randomness concerning a specific drug or dietary regimen

Some common themes emerge in this debate. We will review and discuss these based on available data and scientific sources points.

Why not teach people how to wear a mask properly?

But countries, where people wore masks, had a better result in controlling the epidemic!
Masks can stop transmission of asymptomatic infected individuals and pre-symptomatic.
Mask medical/surgical for health facilities
Medical masks (e.g., N95) and surgical masks are crucial for physicians and nurses' frontline. Protection of workers' health (personal health) infection is crucial to the fight against the pandemic effectively. Medical masks are appropriate for most cautions in the air are in health centers (rather than daily use), and there are dedicated specific guidelines and instructions on how to carry and fit correctly.

Explanation

Surgical masks are primarily designed to protect the environment from the user, while respirators are supposed to protect the user of the situation. However, these differences may not be apparent for non-medical personnel, so here's a brief description.

Surgical masks, also known as face masks or masks procedure, soft devices, folding, disposable creating a physical barrier between the mouth and nose of the user and the environment lose.

N95 respirators are respiratory protection devices designed to achieve a very close fit of the face, which is generally round and adapted to form a seal around the nose and mouth. It is essential to properly keep and wear N95 respirators for them to work effectively.

Medical masks have been shown to have a protective advantage on laboratory surgical masks. However, data are insufficient to determine conclusively whether N95 respirators are superior to surgical masks to protect health workers against communicable acute respiratory infections in healthcare settings.

Surgical masks and medical have strict protocols.

Indeed, studies show that the effectiveness of N95 respirators and surgical masks may be similar for the prevention of influenza. However, this may be because the N95 respirators are uncomfortable and tight, making breathing more difficult, which could lead to more frequent elimination than surgical masks.

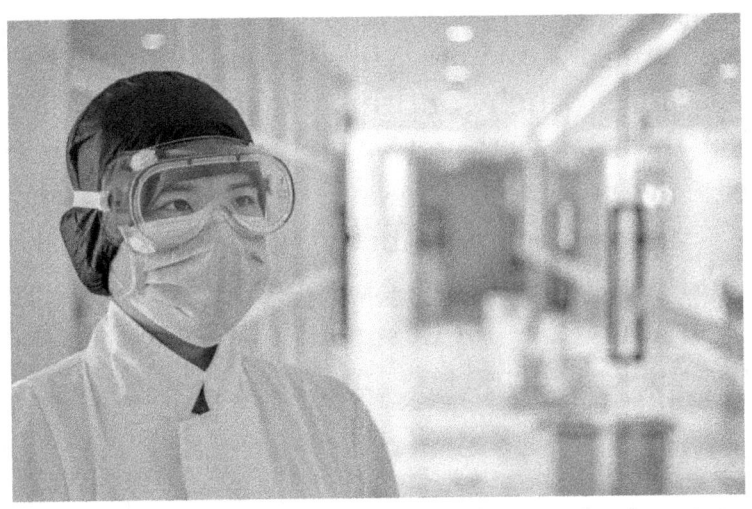

While the N95 respirators may confer superior protection in laboratory studies to obtain a 100% response accession, the systematic use of N95 respirators is less acceptable because they are single uncomfortable in practice. Therefore, these masks cannot be tightly molded to the face, which compromises the benefits of wearing an N95 respirator.

Masks domestic or community settings

If health care workers wear masks, should not the public as well? This debate has led to different policies worldwide.

The World Health Organization (WHO), the Center for Disease Control (CDC), and other public health resources have indicated that the only people who need to wear a face mask are those who are sick or take care of someone who is ill and unable to wear a mask Here, which confirms the above fact: Surgical masks (the easiest to get your hands on) designed to protect an infected person, further their structure enables them to capture body fluids excreted by the oral and nasal cavities (i.e., coughing and sneezing); however, they are not designed to protect the wearer against those infected.

Conversely, N95 masks, which are more challenging to obtain and more expensive to purchase, require specialized training to wear because they must be adequately molded to the wearer's face. Valid, the medical staff receive training and checking that they are adequately equipped.

Many contributing factors determine the effectiveness of masks:

Early use - before the infection is embedded at the location

adequate training - no training, users can not use the cover correctly

proper adjustment - the mask should not allow infectious particles in or outside Hand hygiene - unwashed hands may transfer infectious particles bearer the duration of costumes should be worn most of the time, not just when you go out In short, even if you have an N95 mask, there is a real possibility that this is not done correctly equipped and therefore, ensure optimal protection. So why are so many disagreements about this.

Why are the masks not as useful for the general public?

There is little data regarding masks to reduce the risk of infection at home or in the community.

There is ample evidence that health workers who are adequately trained in the use of masks and are exposed to a large number of infectious respiratory droplets are less likely to be infected.

20/03/2020-Coronavirus-pantryHow to store food for health during panic Coronavirus, However, a systematic review of published data (MacIntyre and Chughtai, 2015) reveals that masks do not prevent or reduce infection within the community when they are the only measure to prevent disease. The reason is that the effectiveness of masks is most likely affected by compliance issues.

There is consistent advice stressing that whether to wear a mask, you should use it appropriately.

This means:

- You should wash your hands before and after use or removal.
- Do not touch the front of it - the part exposed to infection.

- Avoid reaching down to scratch his nose or mouth.
- Use most of the time and discard as soon as it gets wet or damp.
- Otherwise, the use of masks could give a false sense of security.

It shows that compliance with these guidelines decreases in home settings with cover everyday use, which makes using a long-term challenge, In essence, this means that people become laxer about the correct use with time. This is particularly relevant in the current situation because the measures to suppress the spread of COVID-19 are necessary for long periods - not just a few days, but weeks and even months.

N95 masks must be appropriately fitted to work effectively

As noted by many studies, people did not adhere to keep the cover on all the time, simply because the 8uu6masks are uncomfortable. It is a difficult task to comply with all protocols that health workers are trained to routinely and implemented. For this reason, medical masks are recommended for the general public.

Why not teach people correctly use masks?

Teach people to wear a mask is not as easy as you teach them to wash their hands! It is complicated to wear a mask suitable even for health professionals who also are uncomfortable, but they have protocols to ensure compliance.

In addition to the lowest levels of compliance with the protocols of the mask in the home environment, many studies have found that people find less acceptable covers compared to hand hygiene behavior and other non-pharmaceutical interventions Countries using masks had better results in controlling the epidemic.

A recently circulated graph is comparing the mask wear-resistant countries (e.g., South Korea, Japan, Hong Kong, and Singapore) with states that did not ask the general public to wear costumes. The goal? To demonstrate that the wear-resistant mask is instrumental in suppressing COVID-19.

However, it is essential to note that many factors limit the spread of these countries, not only the use of masks. As you can see in the table below, many essential measures undoubtedly had more impact in controlling the spread and break the chain of transmission.

The factors that influence the spread of Covid-19

- strict social distancing quarantine
- cultural etiquette limiting physical contact
- the isolation of sufficient diagnostic tests for mild cases
- Also, several other essential facts have been omitted in this popular graphic. It does not include other countries, such as China, where face masks do not seem to have done much to spread Covid-19.
- Another example is Iceland, which is a remarkably well-controlled disease without the extensive use of face masks to the general public. Moreover, unlike the application, Singapore does not recommend universal covers and limit them to health workers.

The prevention of asymptomatic individuals to infect other

The transmission of symptomatic and asymptomatic individuals was documented pre-COVID for-19, and the viral load is particularly high in the early stages of the disease. This could make a case for wearing a mask as a public health intervention to intercept the transmission link.

DIY masks are not of medical grade protective equipment

However, we must keep in mind that even in

this situation, all the limitations arising from compliance with the cover are still valid. Also, if we assume that everyone is miraculously formed and adheres perfectly to all mask labels, there is still a big problem highlighted by the health authorities of the shortage of global supply chain of personal equipment protection (PPE) in hospitals worldwide.

Health workers have repeatedly reported the insufficient supply of PPE, ranging from gloves and protective gowns to wear goggles and face masks. Anyone who buys a cover for their use is potentially denying a health worker who needs it.

In this situation, there are two possible approaches to solve the problem:

masks home, but this requires technical knowledge of deep physics behind the filtration system tissues and medical masks.
Adhering to the measures based on evidence: washing hands, do not touch your face, physical distancing,

isolation of cases and quarantine.

Consider that this once again. Although a protective mask can reduce the risk of infection, it will not eliminate the risk, especially when the disease is more than one route of transmission. Thus, any mask, no matter how active filtering or the quality of the seal, will have minimal effect if it is not used in conjunction with other preventive measures.

It is premature to assume that the masks protect people Covid-19 itself, and this could put the communities most at risk if you do not follow other strict protocols on how to use this mask and how to stay secure.

CHAPTER 6: PROBLEMS WITH A HOMEMADE MASK

To evaluate the use of a homemade costume, it is useful to know how the right cover (medical and surgical) work. Filtration systems used in modern surgical masks and respirators are considered "fibrous" in Nature: made of a flat, non-woven mat of fine fibers.

Every characteristic of the filtration system, including fiber diameter, porosity (ratio of open space to the fiber), and thickness, plays a role in how well the filter Koleksi particles. In all fibrous filters, three "mechanics" collection mechanisms are in place to capture particles,sq i.e., inertial impaction, interception, and diffusion.

You should wash your hands effectively even with a mask

inertial impaction and interception are the mechanisms responsible for collecting more massive particles, while diffusion is responsible for managing the smaller particles. In some fibrous filters made from fibers charged, an additional tool of electrostatic attraction also operates.

This mechanism helps in the collection of both large and small particles.

This latter mechanism is essential because it increases the particle collection without increasing the breathing resistance. Thus, the mask is not just a simple barrier, and there is more complexity in the cover work correctly, It is also important to note that the CDC, which is a list of homemade masks as an option for health care workers, also provides a choice of five alternatives to be used before switching to DIY:

Excluding health workers with a higher risk for severe illness from COVID-19 from contact with known or suspected COVID-19 patients.
Health workers recover designate (who already have the virus) for the treatment of known or suspected COVID-19 patients.

Use a face shield that covers the entire front (which extends to the chin or below) and the side of the face without a facemask.
Consider using a prudent patient isolation room for patients at risk.
Consider the use of headrests ventilation in hospital beds to reduce exposure.

CDC Guideline has been developed for the use of masks in healthcare settings, so it is essential to understand that homemade masks are considered a last resort. They do not qualify as PPE since their protection capacity is unknown, and CDC urges caution when considering this option.

Many risks associated with cloth masks

cloth masks are commonly used in developing countries, and many non-standard practices regarding their cleaning and reuse have evolved. Most studies on the cloth masks were made before the development of disposable masks. Penetration through tissue is reported high. In one study, it was found that 40-90% of the particles can penetrate the cloth masks.

cloth masks allow more particles
A large prospective study RCT (Macintyre et

al., 2015) showed that water retention, reuse cloth masks, and poor filtration could increase the risk of infection. They showed that the fabric masks have resulted in significantly higher rates of disease than medical masks, and worse than the controls.

fabric masks have given rise to higher infection rates

The virus can survive on the surface of cloth masks. Therefore, self-contamination by repeated use and improper doffing is possible (e.g., cloth mask contaminated pathogen can transfer cover with bare hands of the user).

cloth masks facilitate self-contamination

Although any material can be a physical barrier to infection, if it does not pass matches around the nose and mouth, or the material allows infectious particles to be free through it, it will be useless and dangerous.

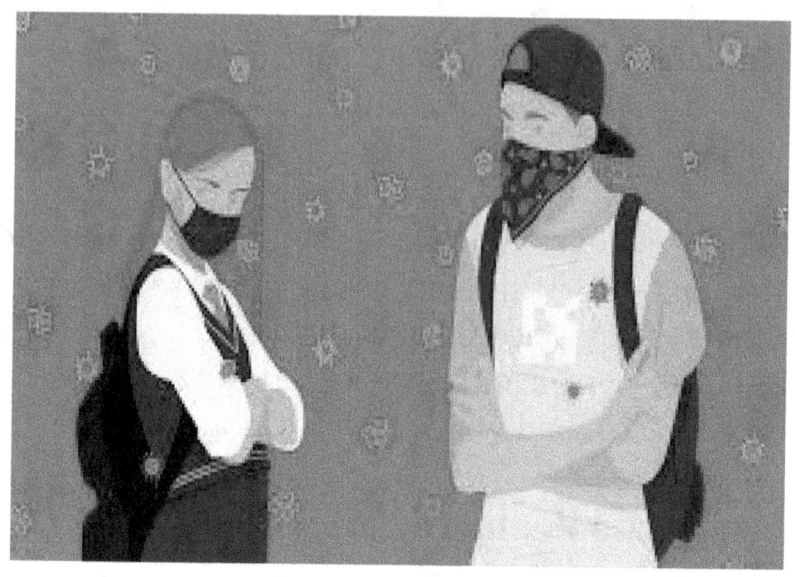

For those who wear a mask to the need, as health workers, regular training and fit testing must be emphasized. Those who choose to wear a mask homemade cleaning requirement must highlight the mask of the change. More importantly, it should be noted so that unnecessary risks are taken lower protective capabilities of a homemade costume.

What is a face mask for virus protection?

better-mask-protection against viruses

Although there are no masks that are specially

designed to protect against the infection alone, you can still find beneficial products that can filter viruses and other airborne particles. If you fear being infected with viruses, then you need to get masks that are approved by NIOSH and gave a rating of N95 or P100. It is those who have proven to be able to stop viruses mostly. You can say what masks are rated N95 or P100 because they are necessary to print detail on the cover itself.

If you do not find any indication of the mask dimension on the surface, or even on the box it came, then it is likely that it is not NIOSH approved at all. Apart from N95 and P100 masks, you can also use quality medical masks with high resistance to fluids. Ideally, they should be those who have resistance at three according to the ASTM standard.

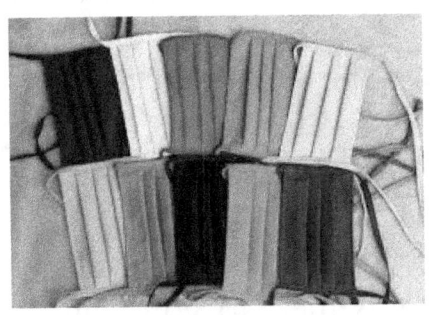

How does it work

Facial masks are air filters that you use on your face. The covers are made of non-woven. These fibers are trapped on the surface of a mesh static electricity charged. This creates a network of tiny holes arranged at random. This filter will provide a physical barrier between the outside air and the nose and mouth.

Masks work by blocking the harmful particles, including viruses, in which air into the nose or mouth. It's like a small network that traps tiny particles in the air, preventing them from getting into the nose and mouth.

The types of virus protection masks

There are many different types of facial masks that you can use to serve as protection against the virus. Here are some of the most popular options:

Medical Mask

This is the most common mask that people are using today. These look like pieces of paper with elastic bands on the sides that hook behind the ears. This form of respiratory protection is based on the filter material, which forms the entire mask.

The colored side of the mask is resistant to the liquid side. This is the part you want to be outside of if you're going to protect yourself from the disease. Now, if you are the one who has the flu, it is necessary
put the colored part of the inside of the mask.

Dust masks are disposable - This is the type of

cover which is generally used by craftsmen like carpenters, drywallers, carpenters, welders, and others who require respiratory protection. Note that these masks look like they are made of stiff paper.

However, the truth is that they are made of fibers which are joined together to create a fine mesh net, thereby preventing liquid and solid particles from getting through. A well as the masks medical/surgical, dust masks can be used only once. After that, then you should properly dispose of it. Never reuse this mask as its effectiveness and will have decreased by much.

Half-face respirators

These are the heavy-duty used for hazardous work environments. These have removable filters that are approved by NIOSH and rated N95 or P100 because they need to block the microscopic airborne irritants to the same asbestos fibers, glass fiber, silica, and others Do these masks be able to defend against viruses? Of course, they could. The only hindrance is that it will be disturbing when leads are out of the workplace. Also, they will be very intolerable to wear a whole sooner or later.

CHAPTER 7: WHY DO YOU NEED A FACE MASK FOR PROTECTION ANTIVIRUS?

The reason you need a face mask is that you can significantly reduce the chances of getting infected with the deadly disease when it comes to the outbreak of the virus. If your nose and mouth with a barrier that prevents aerosols are carriers of the virus to get through, then not be affected by them.

The way the virus is spread through coughing or sneezing of an infected person. The virus is carried in the saliva, and in the limited time that these particles are in the air if another person inhales, there is a good chance that they will become infected with the disease themselves

From now on, the virus is not airborne but has a limited distance you can travel. Besides wearing a mask, you should practice good personal hygiene also. You need to keep your hands clean because you may unknowingly touch a surface covered by the virus. This could put you at risk of touching the eyes, nose, or mouth with the virus, which leads to you getting the dangerous disease.

When it is your health that is on the line, you must ensure that the mask you buy can provide you with enough care and protection you need. Here are some things you should keep an eye on to purchase a good cover designed to protect you from viruses:

Stability

The first and foremost reason why you are considering buying masks is that you want to protect yourself and your family from being infected with the deadly virus circulating now. That is why, whenever possible, you should get one that is listed in the approved face mask CDC.

Now, it is understandable that people due to panic buying masks in bulk, most things in the CDC's list could be out of stock. If that is the case, then you should get one that is NIOSH approved and rated N95 or P100. These were most likely to block harmful particles in the air, which also happens to include bacteria.

Comfort - Many might think that comfort is not essential for masks, but it is. Even if you are dead serious about wearing your protective mask if, after an hour, it becomes unbearably uncomfortable under the cover, you will not want to pay more.

This could also be the time when you start to get complacent and more prone to infection. A good mask should be so light you'll forget you're wearing after a while. Here too

should be a way for your exhaled breath out of the cover.

This will prevent the inside of the mask to warm and soft. Moreover, it will save you from recycling your breath, which means you will not breathe in the carbon dioxide you just exhale.

Another factor that can contribute to a level of comfort is the head strap used to hold the mask in place. It should be neither too tight nor too loose. It should provide just enough elasticity to keep the cover in place.

Type mask

As mentioned above, many types of covers can be used to protect against viral infection, and levels of protection they offer also vary.

First, there is what we call as the disposable mask. You can buy this disposable type bulk for pennies each. The level of protection they offer is moderate at best, but if you're in a bind, you can expect that it is already working.

CHAPTER 8: THERE IS ALSO THE N95 MASKS OR REUSABLE P100.

These masks are much better protection against

viruses, but they are a little more expensive. Also, you can use them for more than a day, but not by much. Most reusable masks can be used for about three days or until they get too dirty.

There are also bulky half-face respirators. They are those used by professional traders when they have to work in hazardous environments, such as when they must break down the walls and ceilings containing asbestos or must work with the delicate glass fiber.

Although these will give you more than enough protection, which is challenging to use in public and will also be very alarming to others.
Fit - Regardless of the type chosen, a good mask should fit properly on your face. There should be no space along the sides that allow outside air to enter into the cover. This contradicts the goal of bringing the mask in the first place.

An excellent way to know if there is a gap between the mask and the face is wearing glasses with the cover. If the windows fog at the exhaling, there is a gap around the mask's nose.
To close this gap, pinch the metal band on the mask found on the bridge of the nose so it will take the shape of your nose. This will close the gap at the top of the cover.

Duration of use - Medical masks and dust

masks are usually only just one use. Medical covers are only usable for three to four hours. If you feel that the inside is already wet, then you need to dispose of it immediately.

There are also reusable masks. Generally, are those exhale valves. Depending on the brand and the brand, you will often find a good cover for at least three days to a week.

Then there is the professional level. These are masks that can be reused indefinitely. Simply replace the filter cartridges once they are full. Most of the covers fall into this category are large and bulky and would look weird when used in public.

However, you can also find some of them seem regular facial masks but small cartridge filters/pads.

Cost and quantity - If you are thinking of buying a disposable type mask, you should ensure you get the most out of your money, literally. Disposable masks, such as medical masks, are cheap enough unless the seller jacks up the price due to increased demand, which is certainly unethical.

This does not mean you should get the cheapest out there. It is because you cannot be sure of its quality. You should buy masks that are sure of massively quality. This is because they are usually cheaper that way. A box of 100 masks can be much more expensive than a six-pack. When you do the math, you will find that the box 100s has a much lower unit price. Besides, the shape of things at this time, you may need to use facial masks for a long time, so it is best to have a lot in stock.

If you want something that is on the side of high strength and is worthy of being put in the survival kit of any person, payable over a hundred dollars for a full-face or half-face respirator.

Care and maintenance

If you are using disposable masks, you should immediately dispose of them at the end of the day. Never reuse disposable masks, especially surgical masks.

Also, if your medical mask gets wet, dispose of it immediately and use a new one instead. Another thing to consider is that when you start to feel that the cover is already humid, it is no longer usable.

Typically, all disposable masks, regardless of whether medical or dust masks need to be discarded after a day of use. Reuse is likely to get you infected if any viruses are trapped on the surface of the cover.

You must have masks properly. First, place them in a plastic bag, tie it, and put it back in the tray of hazardous waste. On the other hand, if you have a reusable mask, you should still have filter cartridges spending correctly and adequately clean the cover itself.

Most reusable masks are made of silicone, so they are straightforward to clean. There is only wiped with a solution made of equal parts of water and alcohol, and you're done.

CONCLUSION

This booklet us know the usefulness of wearing and non-wearing of a mask. Although it may be beneficial when the carrier is adequately trained on how to use and adheres to all other mask labels, there are other measures to protect against the spread of the virus and the risk behind it. Wash your hands, do not touch your face, and practice physical distancing.

www.ingramcontent.com/pod-product-compliance
Lightning Source LLC
Chambersburg PA
CBHW070318220526
45465CB00004B/1896